Axis of Interplanetary Vibrations
Clinical Studies in Medical Astrology

@Copyright Dr. Bobbi Anne White
Smashwords Edition
January 3, 2012

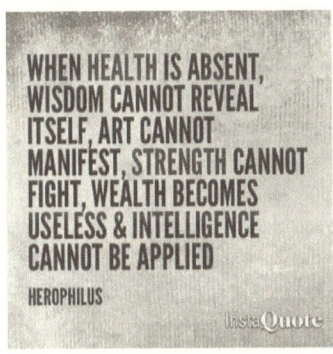

Herophiles 300 B.C.
"No illness which can be treated by diet should be treated by any other means."
Moses Maimonides (1135-1204 A.D.)

This book is dedicated to my loving parents, Allen and Florence White, who have been steadfast with me through all my trials and tribulations. Furthermore, it is dedicated to my spiritual masters of the Madhva Gaudiya Sampradaya in Nabadwip Dham who helped me to surrender to these trials and tribulations as challenges in articulating my true purpose in life. Additionally, I wish to thank other members of Sri Caitanya Saraswat Math for their timely support, in particular, Sriman Narahari das.

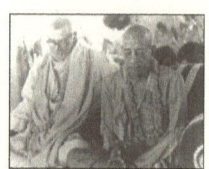

"You may be the lord of all you survey,
but you are a lord in a cremation ground."
Bhakti Raksak Sridhar dev Goswami
I would like to acknowledge that the real inspiration for this book comes from the loving guidance of my divine gurus. Therefore, this book is dedicated to my divine

master, Srila Bhakti Sridhar dev Goswami and his dearmost servitor, Srila Bhakti Sundar Govinda Swami of Nabadwip Dham, India. I pray that the information in this book will inspire the public to take Preventative Medicine more seriously. However, it is only by understanding one's individual Karma that one can truly prevent chronic, degenerative dis-ease. Therefore, I wish to acknowledge the inspiration that I received from the Astrological writings of the Dr. Jagannath Rao and, of course, the late B.V. Raman.

It will not come as any surprise to astrologers that the conjunction of certain planets will lead to spiritual imbalances and, subsequently, chronic physical and mental dis-eases. However, it does come as a surprise to the general public, and it is specifically, the general public I wish to reach. It is through the application of alternative therapeutic lifestyles changes, especially diet and the creation of sacred spaces, that healing on the spiritual plane takes place. These subtle changes lead to healing on the physical plane, because the material manifestation is dependent on the spiritual, not the other way around. Today, of course, we are in the middle of a medical revolution inspired by practitioners who are genuinely interested in Preventative Medicine. Dean Ornish, M.D. has mapped out his alternative regime for reversing coronary heart disease. He reminisces about his encounter with Swami Satchiananda in Dallas: the Swami said "Nothing can bring you lasting happiness and inner peace-but you have it already, you just have to quiet down your mind and body to experience it." In his critique of the present day health care system, Dr. Ornish says "the current health care system, which a disease care system, has de facto reasoning: if you don't have insurance or a lot of money, you don't have very good access to medical care."

Of course, in India, it is no surprise that gem therapy in conjunction with lifestyle modifications, leads to the creation, and maintenance, of good health. These practices stem from common knowledge of astrological principles in each person's life, starting from the moment the child enters life. Even Hippocrates, the father of Modern Medicine, is quoted as saying that: "one who is a doctor and not an astrologer is a Fool." Quite often, in the astrological chart, one is able to detect transient vs. chronic dis-ease patterns. It is my prayer that the American public will be more aware of the contribution that Medical Astrology has in reducing the suffering of mankind. It is an accurate and diagnostic tool: the **horo"scope"**, in addition to the **stetho"scope"**, both providing critical insight into patterns of health/dis-ease at birth: every Indian has his/her astrological chart constructed at birth. There is a certain calculated chart, the Dwadasamsa chart, or one-twelfth divisional chart, derived mathematically from the original natal chart, that is diagnostic of dis-ease patterns.

In this book, I will be citing many clinical examples and therapies for clinical practice. Many of these cases were diagnosed without seeing the patient, just from the birth data. There are many cases of mental, as well as physical diseases that are diagnosable from the natal chart. Obviously, if the natal chart documented at birth, then Preventative measures, such as diet, lifestyle modifications and gem therapy can be utilized immediately. Gem therapy should be discussed, since very little is known about this in the United States. Vibrations sent out by the planets affect the physical, structural body. If the planets are well situated at birth, then good effects will ensue for the living entity who has taken birth at that specific time and place. Otherwise, if the planets are badly situated, then evil results will ensue. Also, if "enemy" planets are conjoined, then the living entity will suffer physically, mentally, or emotionally. One of the chief diagnostic clues of cancer and other degenerative, chronic dis-eases is the conjunction of Saturn and the

Sun, whatever house contains these "aspecting" planets will "localize" the disease. Each of the twelve houses also governs a certain part of the body, and each planet also has an effect on different structures/divisions of the human anatomy.

It is also possible to detect certain "mind-sets" from an understanding of the position of the Dragon's Head and the Dragon's Tail (Rahu and Ketu). This determination will be of assistance in helping the patient/client to focus on his/her life mission, and may enable the individual to understand spiritual forces that may be causing distress. It is an understanding of how "distress" can be a motivating factor for change that is important in life counseling. Therefore, what may be acceptable for a 28 year old will probably not be acceptable for a 45 year-old, because at the latter age, one's "spiritual" mission will come into focus. The placement of the Dragon's Head can also be diagnostic of chronic separative dis-eases.

The conjunction of Mercury and Saturn, or Saturn's 3rd or 10th aspect on Mercury will also be predictive of central nervous system dysfunction and can lead to Stress syndromes, including insomnia and chronic depression. The aspect of Saturn on the Moon leads also to chronic depression, but more emotional in nature. The coupling of the nervous system and emotional depression can lead to major Psychotic illnesses, including Manic Depression, Paranoid Schizophrenia, and Bipolar Personality. Variations of these "genetic (chemical) imbalances," when coupled with difficult planetary transits can precipitate clinically manifest situations. According to B.V. Raman, there are eight astrological points to consider the "native" insane. Let's observe a severe clinical case of mental/emotional imbalance/insanity.

Just a word about this latter point, when taking a Medical History, there will usually be denial of any depression, etc., especially, of course, in teenagers or early twenty year olds, since there may not have been any "precipitating" circumstances, i.e., planetary transits. That is why this diagnostic system has an advantage, because at that point, the physician can simply recommend gem therapy or lifestyle modifications, since these do not entail any loss of personal self-esteem, or chemical intervention (medication.) These latter types of intervention usually come when the nervous/emotional system has become so debilitated and the person is so "out-of-control", that he/she presents a danger to him/herself or to society. And, of course, when on medication, the persona is stigmatized as well.

Of course, in any scientific discourse, delineation of the clinical parameters, collection procedures is a basic consideration and since we hope to have an impact on the medical community here in the states and Canada, I will take the time to explain. First of all, all diagnoses were made by telephone, with no other information other than a birth date, a birth time and a place of birth: basic astrological input. Birth time is often unknown, but can be assessed by an acute astrologer who knows the art of "muhurta", or the effect of the rising sign on the query. If the diagnosis was for a person, age 27-28, many incipient signals might be present, but the full-blown symptomatology would probably not be present. If in the age group 39-45, the person might already be in treatment. The reason for this, well known in astrological circles is the "maturation" of the planets (James Braha). In some early-detected cases of mental abnormality, such as ADD or Manic Depression, there might be two or more astrological imbalances in place for the patient, and, in these cases he/she was already treated by medication. The planetary position, conjunctions, etc., were taken from "Raman's 110 Year Ephemeris of Planetary Positions." (you may also use a new free software Junior-jyotish) The full

astrological, sidereal charts will be found in the appendix. Without any previous history, the diagnosis, diagnoses were made on the basis of astrological delineations.
Furthermore, although major involvement of the bones, central nervous system, internal organ system, emotive system, reproductive system was anticipated from the astrological delineation, the specific Latin diagnoses, such as Cystic Fibrosis, Crohn's disease, etc. might not be deduced, unless there was a genetic pattern. Additionally, of course, these patients would usually be diagnosed in conventional medicine, only when the disease has already caused major destruction (in its degenerative stage) or if there were a genetic, familial occurrence. Therefore, I would like to propose a slightly different conceptuality, since, with Astrology, early detection is possible, affording the possibility of conscious alterations in diet, gem therapy and lifestyle modifications. to alter substantially the clinical course of the dis-ease.

In this chapter, I would like to talk more about an alternative medical paradigm, quoting Bill Moyers: "we do need a new medical paradigm that goes beyond body parts medicine, and not only for the patient's sake. At a time, when the cost of health care is skyrocketing, the potential impact of mind/body medicine is considerable." In my own interaction with friends, family and the public, I have seen how the mind/body axis, if inherently weak, will lead subsequently to physical symptoms, not only in deteriorating internal organs, but also in pre-disposing the patient to accidents from rash behavior. There has been much recent evidence, of course, in the field of psychoneuroimmunology to substantiate the claim that one's emotional health alters one's immune system. Dr. David Spiegel says: "health care is more than just physical intervention..." Dr. Eisenberg of Harvard University introduced Dr. Xie (on <u>Dr. Eisenberg's tour Of Bejing Medical University with Bill Moyers</u>) who said "in Chinese medicine the mind and the emotions are closely related to health. For example, disease can be caused by the intensification of any of the seven (7) human emotions-joy, anger, melancholy, brooding, sorrow, fear, and shock."

Therefore, in the examination of a child's astrological chart, weaknesses and pre-disposing factors are considered to create an optimum environment for each child and to reduce the negative impact of malefic vibrations that lead to physical, emotional and mental dis-ease.

According to Dr. Jagannath Rao, each planet has a jurisdiction and an inherent ability to produce disease. I might add, that it is the mal-placed and/or fallen position of these planets that allows them to manifest dis-ease, rather than health. Dr. Rao points out:

The afflicted Sun causes weak eyesight, headaches, and disturbances of circulation, weakness of bone, baldness, hyperirritability, and fevers. The afflicted Moon causes dis-eases of the uterus, dropsy, skin dis-eases, pleurisy or tuberculosis, menstrual disorders, mental aberration, anemia, serous effusions, nervousness. Afflicted Mars causes blood dis-eases, tissue breakage, fevers, burns, mental aberrations, timidity when in debilitation or certain houses, irritability, wounds, eruptions, epilepsy, tumors, etc.

Afflicted Mercury causes mental dis-eases, highly-strung nerves, nervous breakdowns, neuromas, leuco-dermas, excessive sweating, impotence, vertigo, sensitiveness, and deafness. Afflicted Venus causes venereal diseases, sensitiveness, carbuncles, diabetes, stricture urethra, stones in bladder or kidney, parotitis, euphoria, lacrimal troubles, cataract and weakness of sexual organs.

Afflicted Jupiter causes jaundice, diseases of the liver, vertigo, laziness, general lassitude, chronicity of dis-eases, disease of the gall bladder, sleeping sickness anemias, idiosyncrasies. Debilitated Saturn causes paralysis, insanity, chronicity, of dis-ease, cancer and other tumors, elephantiasis, idiocy and glandular dis-eases. Afflicted Rahu causes hiccough, slowness of action, clumsiness, intestinal diseases, insanity, leprosy, ulcers, general debility, boils, eclampsia, varicose veins, disease of spleen and adrenals. Afflicted Ketu causes intestinal worms, epidemics, eruptive fevers, low blood pressure, deafness and defective speech.

CLINICAL CASES

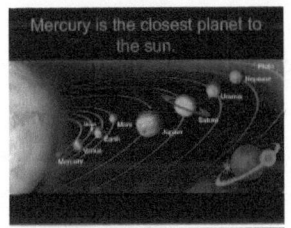

Mercury.

(usually involves the central nervous system with a psychological component.)

Barbara T. born 11/12/1950 10:30 AM This native had a Sun-Saturn conjunction in Virgo, a house owned by Mercury. So, not only did she had chronic physical problem dealing with her central nervous system, but also Fibromyalgia and Cystic Fibrosis which is described as "an inherited disease of the exocrine, affecting the pancreas, respiratory system and sweat glands." (Merck) In this very extensive clinical case, we can see that not only is Saturn conjunct with the Sun, but it is also throwing its 7th aspect on Jupiter and its 3rd aspect on Mars, Mercury and Venus. Therefore, the effects on the pancreas (Jupiter), on the CNS (Mercury), the exocrine system (Venus) and the muscular system (Mars). All these aspects are deleterious.

Lydia T, born 7/30/1981. This native is the daughter of the previous native, Barbara, and has already been diagnosed as manic-depressive. Saturn is throwing its 10th aspect on Mars, which is conjunct with Mercury. Saturn is also conjunct with Jupiter, so the pancreatic effects will be noted as well. Thus, Mercury has the aggressive impulses of

Mars, as well as the chronic aspect of Saturn, leading to the diagnosis of Manic-Depression. (According to J.N. Bhasin, dispositors carry the influence of planets which are situated in their domains (rasis.) Additionally, the Sun and the Moon are both conjunct with the Dragon's head (Rahu), causing paranoia.

Machela C. born 8/15/1941. This native presented with Sciatica, which was gleaned from her chart. Here, Saturn is throwing its 3rd aspect on the conjunction of the Sun and Mercury. Therefore, the dis-ease has both physical and nervous components. Sciatica, of course, is classified as "nerve root dysfunction of the buttock and posterolateral thigh and calf. There may be large lesions in the lumbosacral region involving the many roots of the cauda equina, producing bilateral radicular symptoms in the lower extremities, as well as impaired sphincter and sexual functions, due to the involvement of the sacral region." (Merck) The specific location of the nerve dysfunction can be determined by the most "malefic" planet, which, in this case, is Mars, since it is carrying the indirect weight of Saturn and is also conjunct with Ketu in the house owned by Jupiter, in the constellation of Pisces, which area deals with the lower extremities.

Norman L. birthdate 4/21/1961, 12:39 PM, Illinois. In this chart, Saturn is throwing its 3rd aspect on Mercury and Mars is throwing its' aggressive aspect on the Moon, which is badly placed in the 12th house of loss, and Mars' 8th aspect is simultaneously on Saturn. Therefore, Saturn's aspect on Mercury is also carrying the aspect of Mars. Norman is a well known psychiatric patient. His diagnosis is Manic-depressive and he is also extremely violent, if not on his meds. He currently takes Lithium and Respiridol and also follows a strict vegetarian diet and practices yoga. He was first diagnosed during a major Saturn *dasa* (period), sub-period Mars, when he was 21 years old, and has been in and out of hospitals since then. Considering the severity of his dis-ease he does moderately better than others with the same diagnosis: he manages his own finances and housing.

Ashley M. birth date 8/30/1968 @ 7:30 AM Miami. This patient is patient from the Crisis Center of Dade County, and has been treated after an apparent suicide. This case is more indirect and the subtleties are acting indirectly by the placement of Mars in the domain (rasi) of the Moon. Also, according to Bhasin's dispositor theory, Mars is carrying the influence of the fallen Saturn. This patient was diagnosed after his second suicide attempt in 1993. He started taking herbs for depression and continued his Astanga Yoga (breathing exercises), but discontinued his therapy and ended up in the Crisis Center twice in 1997. In spite of the sincere attempts of alternative practitioners, he does not accept advice. Astrologically this arrogance can be noted by a certain "Vaidhriti Yoga", which is simply sum of the Sun and the Moon's position. There are 27 such Yogas

(B.V. Raman) These Yogas are important in Muhurta astrology, which allows the astrologer to select an auspicious day to begin a project, or avoid a bad one. This yoga can also be noted as part of the native's natal chart.

Margaret P. birthdate 7/13/71 @ 2:30 PM Boston. This native studied yoga early in life and also became a vegetarian. It will be noted that in her astrology chart, there are severe disturbances in her emotional and CNS. This is due to the influence of Saturn's 3rd aspect to Mercury, which is also conjunct Ketu; additionally, Mars is throwing its full aspect on Mercury. Furthermore, Saturn is casting its 10th aspect on the Moon, which is also bearing the indirect dispositor's burden of Ketu. Additionally, since the Moon is devoid of planets on either side of it, there is a manifestation of *Kemadruma Yoga*, which makes one feel lonely. She was prescribed a pearl in India and an emerald and functioned very well, until recently after the birth of her first child. At that time, she had a manic-depressive episode and sought out the advice of a therapist. The psychiatrist wanted her to put her child in foster care and start medication. However, a Reiki healer and a naturopath recommended moving to a more supportive environment. (Her husband had to travel for work) So the entire episode acted as a catalyst for change, rather than institutionalization and medication. Effects, therefore, were moderate and transient, since she decided to remove herself from the stressful, materialistic society and took shelter in a more supportive environment. Therefore, the gem therapy and increased flexibility therapy contributed successfully to her avoidance of institutionalization. Of course, any astrologer would note that the saving grace in her chart is that the lagnesh (lord of the 1st house) is in the 9th house of fortune, religion and good luck. This astrological placement gives her a disposition to listen to spiritual authorities.

Ajah G. birthdate 8/29/92 Sickle cell anemia: he was a descendant of an Afro-American football legend. Sickle cell tends to be confined to the Afro-American community. In the chart, Mars is throwing its' 4th aspect on Jupiter and Saturn is aspecting the Sun-Mercury conjunction. Since the Sun planet is in charge of the functions of the bone and since, of course, RBC's contribute to the health of the bony structure, we could predict chronic involvement. The aspect of Mars on Jupiter also plays a part, in that the spleen function also plays a critical part in the production of hemoglobin. Since the cause of death, according to Merck are "inter-current infections (especially tuberculosis), multiple pulmonary emboli. "It would seem relevant that the aspect of Saturn on the Sun-Mercury conjunction takes place in the Kalaparusha domain usually considered the "lung-chest area." (Rao)

Obviously, in cases where there is severe depression, the patient may decide to self-medicate and, hence, bring about other medical problems. Such was the case with Cornelia, birthdate 8/15/1962 @ Las Vegas. Here we observe that Saturn and the Nodes are directly aspecting the Sun owned by the Moon (Cancer). This combination in itself will predispose to pulmonary difficulties. However, the patient is accelerating his cocaine use.

The same conjunctions of Saturn and Mercury can give unparalleled research abilities, even Einstein genius. (ref: James Braha), but, due to the heavy stress on the CNS, will eventually predispose one to melancholy and insomnia. We noticed this in the chart of a brilliant student, Heidi, whose birthdate is 11/30/1972 @ 5:09 AM Ma. She suffers from chronic depression. Myasthenia gravis: this is, according to Merck, "a disease characterized by chronic muscular fatigue and weakness, occurring chiefly in muscles innervated by the cranial nerve." This is Judy, birthdate 1/14/1931 @ 3PM, Pa. Mars is *neecha* (fallen) and is directly aspecting the Sun. Saturn is conjunct Mercury and is also aspecting Jupiter. This again, in such a complicated disease, causes numerous afflictions. Emphysema, defined by Merck as an "irreversible, generalized airway obstruction...caused by chronic inflammatory reaction at the alveolar level." Merck theorizes that "anything which...allows low-grade inflammatory reactions to develop" is a precursor to the dis-ease. The patient here is Rick W. birthdate 9/9/1958 KY. Notice the double malefic effect of Mars, which is carrying the aspect of Saturn on the Sun-Mercury conjunction. Therefore, even though his dis-ease is correlated with his employment in the coal mines of Kentucky, there is still a genetic predisposition. Furthermore, there is a psychological component of depression.

Central Nervous System Poisoning: This is a case of a Desert Storm veteran, who is manifesting symptoms of "nervousness." His name is Howard A. birthdate 12/16/1955, Ala. There is an ominous quad-junction of Saturn-Sun-Mercury-Rahu. The latter planetary involvement (Rahu) indicates the etiology, namely poisoning. This is well known in astrological circles. His claim is pending with the VA and he has severe spinal symptoms, which, in his case, will progress. We have recommended gem therapy and a vegetarian diet for detoxification.

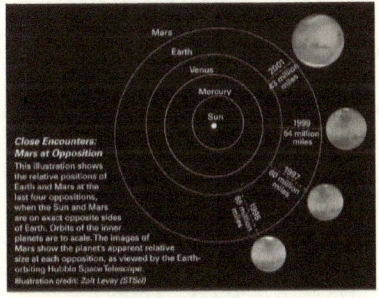

Sun-Mars Conjunction

The next planetary conjunction is noted invariably as an early warning sign that the patient may be suffering from low self-esteem, and that the patient may have suffered from physical abuse, or may be predisposed to accepting abuse. Aside from the psychological effects, there are also physical symptoms and I would like to present one. There is an example of one celebrity with this conjunction in his chart, Gianni Versace, the designer, who was stalked and assassinated in Miami Beach, July 15, 1997. In fact, he was shot between the eyes. "The shooter fired twice, striking the victim once in the center of his face to the right of his nose, and once in the left side of his neck, just below the left ear." (autopsy report Miami Beach Police) His birthdate is 12/2/1946 @ 1:30 PM, Reggio di Calabria, Italy. Mars-Ketu is conjunct the Sun, the *significator* of the left eye and the same conjunction is also throwing its 4th aspect on the Moon, the significator of the right eye. Not only is the Sun conjunct malefic Mars, it is also conjunct Ketu, which, of course, acts like Mars, a fact well known to astrologers. The shot to the neck is from the 7th aspect of Mars-Ketu on the second house of the Kalaparusha, which is Taurus, which governs the head-neck region. So, assassination was just waiting to happen. Proper counseling would have assisted him in changing his karma, to avoid this tragedy. Unfortunately, this did not happen. Given this understanding, he may have altered his lifestyle.

Additionally, this particular condition (Sun-Mars) will invariably lead to low self-esteem and/or, in many cases, physical abuse, assassination of the Native. You will see it also in the chart of President Abraham Lincoln and Prime Minister Benazir Bhutto, who could not be protected from it by 15,000 troops. There is also a case of Multiple Sclerosis that involves this combination. Other planets, Jupiter and Venus, are conjunct with the Sun; this whole tri-junction is aspected by Mar's full 7th aspect and by Saturn's 10th aspect. The native's, Lynn, birthdate is 9/2/1956 @10:57 PM. Several of her organ systems were endangered. Merck describes Multiple Sclerosis as "de-myelination and cortico-spinal involvement.

There is toxic muscular weakness and 'intention tremor.' There is apathy, lack of judgment, emotional lability and reactive depression. In later stages, there are convulsive seizures." It should be noted that one of the early symptoms in retro-bulbar optic neuritis (partial blindness and pain in one eye) It is common knowledge in astrological circles, that the Sun governs the left eye and the Moon the right. They are the "luminaries." Therefore, the Sun-Mars conjunction may lead to vision problems as well. This may seem all very speculative, however, it is to be remembered that a diagnosis of problems was obtained over the phone without a Medical history. It should also be remembered that a diagnosis is usually given in the later stages of the illness. There is a major organ involvement, including the CNS, cranial nerves, cerebral nerves and paresthesis, autonomic nervous system (bladder involvement leading to incontinence.) Therefore, it might be postulated that the aspect of Mars and Saturn on this "tri-junction of Jupiter-Sun-Venus" is predictive of such a debilitating dis-ease. Additionally, a there is the aspect of the Nodes, as well, carried by conjunction with malefic Saturn. Each one of these planets is responsible for maintaining different parts of the body through a specific vibration. I will speak more about this later, in the discussion of Gem Therapy as a Preventative modality to be considered in the alteration of detected dis-ease patterns.

Another Sun-Mars involvement occurred with a friend's son, whose astrological profile was unknown to us until he had a heart attack while playing basketball on 10/2/1997 (Vaidhriti Yoga). Gato's birthdate is 10/3/1981 @ 7:30 PM NY. It will be noted that Mars is in the Sun's domain (Simha), providing another Sun-Mars conjunction. From early childhood, he has been on a medical alert due to a septal atrial defect. However, with the onset of his "teens", he departed from medical advice and played basketball. It might be conjectured that his lack of self-esteem predisposed him to jeopardizing his life, since he had been advised extensively both by his parents and physician to avoid strenuous physical activity. He has been a vegetarian since birth and a practitioner of yoga. He has since recovered the use of his extremities, although for one month he was paralyzed. One might wonder what his chances might have been, had he not been on a vegetarian diet. Obviously he failed to follow the strict regime that a septal defect mandated, and even a vegetarian diet will not override those strict limitations of heavy athletic participation.

Another client asked me to look at her chart, and I suspected a heart defect. Amy's birthdate is 6/24/1979 @ 4:08 AM, Fl. she responded that she was diagnosed with a septal defect as a child. I referred her to a Mental Health Clinic, since she suffers from low self-esteem and depression. Mars is throwing its 4th aspect on Saturn, which is in the domain of the Sun (Simha.) Again, note the involvement of the Nodes, situated in Simha (Leo). These additional aspects increase the severity of the symptoms. There is another case with the Sun-Mars conjunction and with the additional component of Saturn's 3rd aspect. This patient is being treated for psoriasis and chronic depression with lithium by allopathic practitioners. Barbara's birthdate is 6/11/1966 Ca. I referred her for a naturopathic evaluation, considering that she is really suffering from stress and emotional factors, due to a twelve year abusive relationship. Psoriasis is described by Merck as " a common chronic and recurrent disease characterized by dry, well-circumscribed, silvery, scaling papules and plaques of various disease...the cause is unknown." Psoriasis is, of course, a stress-related disease. According to Helmut Christ, M.D. of West Germany, "it has now that psoriasis is not a skin disorder, but instead a metabolic disturbance which is triggered by environmental or stressful conditions."

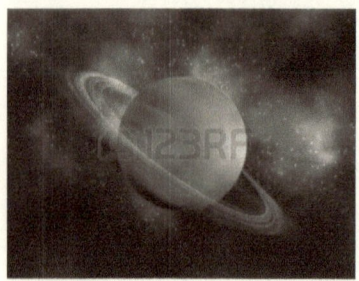

SATURN

When the planet Saturn is debilitated, or as we call it, "angry" it has the power to inflict serious medical conditions, often chronic. It is, of course, considered a highly malefic planet. Whenever Saturn aspects the Sun, there will be a chronic health problem. It is important to consider the house placement of Saturn, whether it is in a "friendly" house, whether it is debilitated and also what "benefic" planets it may be aspecting, because those planets also are related to the different anatomical features of the body. One important thing to consider is also whether there may be a "neechabanga" yoga, which is a correction, if you will, of the dangerous effects noted in the natal chart. For example if Saturn is in the same position in the Navamsa chart, there will be a "correction." If the "angry" planet is located in the early (zero) degrees in the natal chart, it could be considered "void", or rather impotent. The 12th Divisional Chart, Dwadasamsa, is very important in the complete evaluation of the medical prospects of the native. For example, if you only considered the natal chart of Abraham Lincoln, you would miss the clear indications of his being assassinated, namely the Sun conjunct Mars and Saturn.

To sum up, there is ample evidence to conclude that the aspect of Mars, either directly by aspect, or indirectly by association, will pre-dispose the Native to low self-esteem and, hence, poor judgment, known as the "vulnerable personality." These observations are in line with the previous statement of Dr. Xie to Dr. Eisenberg that "disease can be caused by the intensification of any of the seven human emotions- joy, anger, melancholy, brooding, sorrow, fear and shock." In her book, <u>Anatomy of the Spirit</u>, Dr. Carolyn Myss, also indicated that unresolved emotions result in wounds and disease, appearing in any of the seven chakras. Asthma and inferiority complex: Lasandra, birthdate 7/28/1978, Tn. This is an overweight, asthmatic patient who also suffers from an emotional disorder. Of course, it is well known that emotional triggers are the source of asthmatic attacks and Lasandra has been counseled extensively in this regard. Additionally, she might also wear a ruby to enhance the power of the Sun.

The house placement of malefic planets, in Virgo, the 6th house, according to Kalaparusha is indicative of severe chronic disease. Kalaparusha simply means that each of the twelve houses governs certain parts of the body. Virgo, also being the 6th house, in order from Aries, is even more involved in health matters. There are two people I would like discuss, whose charts are rather notable for the severity of their illnesses. The first one is actually my father, Allen, birthdate 9/21/1917, Ma. Saturn and Mars are conjunct and throwing their combined aspect (3rd on the Mercury-Sun conjunction in Mars). After serving in WW II, he suffered from chronic ulcerative colitis and had surgery in 1956 for a complete colestomy.

The second is Gudrun, who was a homeless woman we helped. Her birthdate is 2/15/1952 @ 2 AM, Germany. She suffers from Crohn's Disease (according to Merck, Crohn's is non-specific granulomatous inflammatory disease usually affecting the lower ileum, but often involving the colon. She had just been released from a hospital, where she underwent a partial colonic resection. Notice the position of Saturn in Virgo. which is also throwing its full 7th aspect on Jupiter, thus causing other internal organic deficiencies. I recommended a vegetarian diet and exercise, but she disappeared. During the time we knew her, she made quite a point of being a Christian, but since she is from Germany, possibly she wanted to avoid the notion of being Jewish, since Crohn's does have a familial tendency amongst Jews. She has been in the U.S. without papers and has been living on the streets, so I also speculate that she may have a persecution complex. Obviously, Germany would be in a better position to provide for Gudrun, especially since she has many medical needs. I make that statement because Saturn is conjunct the Moon and that conjunction does "cause" the person to fabricate stories (Kaput Yoga).

The following is a case of a brain tumor in a child, caused by the aspect of Saturn on the ruler of the Kalaparusha domain. Namely, Saturn is aspecting Mars by its' 10th aspect, which is the ruler of the first Kalaparusha house, Aries. Also, according to the *dispositor* theory, Mercury, conjunct with the Sun in Simha, is acting as Saturn. Furthermore, Saturn is receiving the 4th aspect of Mars. The Native is Sue, birthdate 8/27/1981 @ 8:42 AM. Tx. Recall that in the planetary jurisdiction, afflictions to Mercury result in mental diseases, highly strung nerves, nervous breakdown, neuromas, leucoderma, excessive sweating, impotence, vertigo, sensitiveness, and deafness. Mars and Saturn are in Mercury's houses (Virgo and Gemini), that Mercury thus carries both energies in its conjunction with the Sun planet, leading to brain surgery.

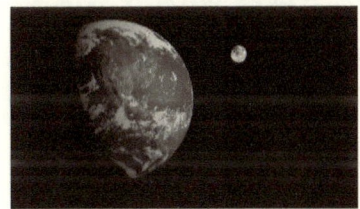

MOON

Emotional depression, reproductive system disorders, asthma, bronchitis

The clinical cases that I will present here have either the Moon heavily afflicted, or the house owned the Moon (Cancer) afflicted. Additionally, another water sign, Scorpio, is frequently sighted in cases involving surgical intervention of the reproductive system. Naomi's birthdate 12/19/1951 @ 1:005 PM, Mn. The Mars-Saturn conjunction is throwing its combined aspect on Scorpio, which is the Kalaparusha house for the reproductive system. Therefore, in a Mars/Saturn "transit", she had a hysterectomy. However, the usual pathology that might be anticipated from the heavy malefic aspect on Mercury is absent, due to her having adopted a strict vegetarian and yoga in her 20's. I would say that she has had several extremely painful experiences, which could have plunged any other less developed individual into a severe depression, such as happened with the following individual. Terry B: birthdate 12/20/1951 @ 4 AM NY. As you might notice, he is just 16 hours younger than the previous case, Naomi. Terry has been a psychiatric patient for some time and takes Lithium. During those 16 hours, the Moon moved from 13 degrees 25 minutes to 21 degrees. One wonders what would have been his outcome if he had taken up lifestyle modifications such as Naomi had. Terry is articulate and artistically inclined, but clinically, being on heavy medications does keep him from making progress in the normal world. It was an amazing revelation to meet a person who is practically a twin of the former yoga teacher. His physical stature is similar as well: they are both tall (6'2").

Raynaud's Disease: Denis, birthdate 1/6/1964 @ 12:05 PM, Ca. Merck describes this as "idiopathic" functional peripheral disorder that may be secondary to an organic dis-ease, and it may be due to "occlusive arterial disease, connective tissue disorder and is most commonly found in young women." However, my diagnosis was given after a preliminary estimation from her chart of secondary effects from the degeneration of internal liver dysfunction. From an analysis of her astrological chart, it can be noted that Mars-Saturn conjunction is fully aspecting Jupiter. Additionally, in my own case I had a paresthesia of the digits that was cured by wearing blue topaz. My birthdate is 4/21/1945 @ 8:30 AM, Va. Note the heavy malefic 3rd aspect of Rahu-Saturn on Jupiter, as well as Mars on Jupiter, by its 4th aspect. Asthma is due to the conjunction of Sun-Saturn in the house owned by the Moon, i.e., Cancer. Megan's birthdate is 8/11/1977, Va. In this case, the young lady was going off to college and was already anticipating the emotional stress involved in that major move. She was already a vegetarian and was aware that asthma had an emotional component.

Melissa is a complicated study. Birthdate is 12/19/1978, Va. She was already being treated for asthma and has borderline thyroid deficiency, but is not being treated. Secondly, she also suffers from low self-esteem. Noticeable in her astrology chart is the aspect of Mars by its 8th aspect on exalted Jupiter (in Cancer) the conjunction of Saturn with the Moon, predisposing towards asthma, and thirdly, the conjunction of Sun-Mars, diminishing her self esteem in relationships. The thyroid deficiency points out the involvement of Rahu, which is conjunct Saturn. (Rahu: hiccough, slowness of action, clumsiness, intestinal diseases, insanity, leprosy, ulcers, general debility, boils, eclampsia, varicose veins, disease of the spleen and adrenals.)

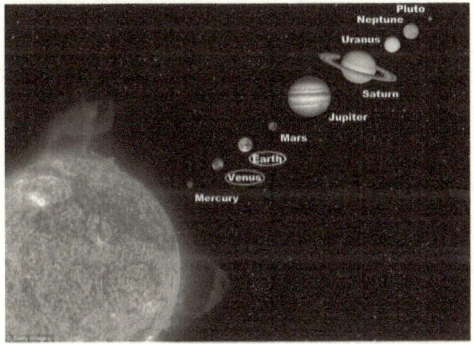

VENUS

Venereal diseases, sensitiveness, carbuncles, diabetes, stricture urethra, stones in bladder or kidney, parotitis euphoria, lacrimal troubles, cataract and weakness of the sexual organs. Venus governs the sexual organs, hence, the name venereal. We have a clinical case, Emma C. birthdate 7/12/1976, NY. Her symptoms were severe, including loss of hair, and a possible breast cyst. Notice that Saturn is conjunct Venus, in the house owned by the Moon (Cancer) and also aspecting directly the Moon. Therefore, her sexual (secondary) organs, as well as her reproductive system were afflicted.

A case of AIDS: Jim, birthdate 6/28/1960. During his 12 year marriage, Jim had numerous extra-marital affairs, that destroyed the marital trust. Now both he and his wife are experiencing symptoms of chronic disease, initially, skin lesions and then progressed into severe depression. Examination of Jim's chart reveals that not only is Saturn conjunct Jupiter, but also Saturn is casting its malefic aspect on the

Sun-Venus conjunction. Jim is in the early stages of AIDS.

As indicated above, afflictions of Venus can also cause kidney stones. This man, Joseph, was just starting to experience "kidney stones". His birthdate is 11/15/1975. Notice that not only is Mars casting its 4th aspect on Venus, but also Saturn is throwing its 3rd aspect as well. At this time, he was just beginning diagnostic testing.

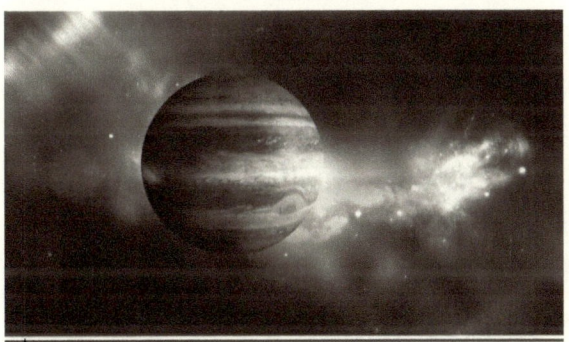

JUPITER

Causes jaundice, dis-eases of the liver, vertigo, laziness, general lassitude, chronicity of dis-eases, dis-eases of the gall bladder, sleeping sickness anemia, idiosyncrasies.

The following is a clinical case of brain tumor behind the left eye in a diabetic patient, Anna, whose birthdate is 6/11/1958, Ma. She was extremely surprised when I asked her if she had a medical problem in the head-neck region. Saturn is aspecting the Sun and Saturn is located in the Kalaparusha area of the head-neck, Taurus. she said that no one in her family knew she had a tumor in the back of her left eye. Examination of her chart reveals several factors: Mars is conjunct the Moon in a house owned by Jupiter. Secondly, Mars is also aspecting Jupiter by its 7th aspect. This Mars-Jupiter opposition is responsible for the organic imbalance in her pancreas. Thirdly, the ominous opposition of the Sun and Saturn. She also has idiopathic back pain and that she frequently could not walk, due to her left leg. (Mars' effect in the Kalaparusha area of Pisces), governing the extremities. She claimed that her doctors could not understand the cause of the idiopathic swelling and disability of the foot. One wonders if the term "idiopathic" more rightly refers to the "idiots" who claim to be the doctors. (As Hippocrates warned.) Furthermore, they had promised to discontinue the insulin, when she lost weight, but they kept putting her off. She also felt that the surgery on her back was useless. Another doctor casually told her that a hysterectomy was next, all part of the schedule. All in all, she had a somewhat familiar pattern of discontent with the "body parts medical" approach. I referred her to Dr. George Duke's book <u>THE GREEN PHARMACY</u> which recommends phytoestrogens for women. Coincidentally, she seemed to be blessed, since her 80 year old father had just given her a blue topaz, which is the gem of choice for an afflicted Jupiter.

Jupiter governs the functioning of the internal organs. Dysfunction: Victoria S: birthdate 10/28/1935, Ma. Notice in her chart that Mars is conjunct Jupiter and that this combined conjunction is throwing its aspect on Saturn, which, in turn is throwing its' aspect on Venus. This leads me to believe that the thyroid imbalance will necessitate the affliction of more than one planet. Since, of course, the thyroid is responsible for growth and metabolism, very often, dysfunction of the thyroid will lead to changes in hormone levels as well, mandating changes in estrogen levels, etc. In a previous complicated case (Melissa, born 12/19/1978) multiple afflictions were noted, especially, Mars 8th aspect on Jupiter.

Another severe case of kidney dysfunction and diabetes Herbert M. 6/9/1950, N.C. Notice that in this case, there are again, several major planetary afflictions, starting with the conjunction of Mars and Saturn in the house owned by the Sun (Leo). this conjunction throws its aspect on the conjunction of Mercury-Sun. Mars and Saturn are also directly aspecting Jupiter. Thus, there is major organ involvement (Jupiter) chronicity, and furthermore, a severe chronic depression.

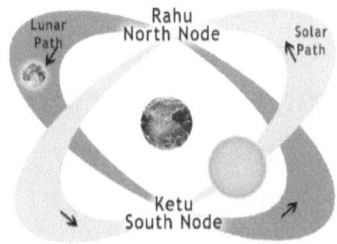

RAHU

Hiccough, slowness of action, clumsiness, intestinal dis-eases, insanity, leprosy, ulcers, general debility, boils, eclampsia, varicose veins, disease of the spleen and adrenals.

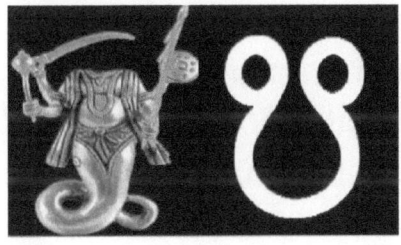

KETU

Intestinal worms, epidemics, eruptive fevers, low blood pressure, deafness and defective speech.

A case of bleeding ulcers. Louise: birthdate 11/6/1953 @ 6 AM, Hi. Notice in her chart, Saturn is conjunct the Sun and the Moon (dark Moon). Furthermore, Ketu is in the house owned by the Moon. According to the dispositor *theory*, the Moon would thus be carrying the Nodal energy into the already severe conjunction of the Sun-Saturn. Additionally, this whole tri-junction is taking place in the Kalaparusha domain of Libra which is in charge of the kidneys and GI area. The Nodes are notorious enemies of the luminaries, the Sun and the Moon. As such, the disease, bleeding ulcers id based on a psychological dimension. According to MERCK: "Stress has been implicated as a commonly occurring precipitating component." Ketu is very often a factor in inducing mental stress, especially if it is associated with one of the luminaries. Obviously, if Ketu is involved by direct conjunction, Rahu will be a contributing factor, by its' 7th aspect.

The following is a case of paralysis, due to brain surgery, and mis-diagnosis. This is Charlie B, birthdate 3/23/44, Md. Here again is the insidious presence of Rahu in the house of a luminary, the Moon, and conjunct exalted Jupiter. Saturn, no doubt has a part to play in this unfortunate scenario, since it is throwing its 3rd aspect on the Rahu-Jupiter conjunction. Since Saturn is also throwing its' 10th aspect on the Moon-Venus conjunction, the house owned by the Moon would be effected. Thus the Rahu-Jupiter conjunction is again carrying the double negative impact of Saturn, according to the "dispositor" theory. The fact that he is bipolar and, hence, misunderstood, also helps us to understand the *karma* of paralysis by misdiagnosis.

Initially, of course, this astrological knowledge was passed down by very learned sages, and is still preserved in the BRIHAT PARASARA HORA SASTRA, because the initial knowledge was passed down originally from "Lord Brahma to (Lord Shiva and his consort

Parvati) and then to the Sage Narada, and from him to Saunaka and then to Parasara who was actually the grandfather of the incarnation of Krsna, Vyasadeva, who is the father of Krsna. The remedies described in the <u>BRIHAT PARASARA HORA SASTRA</u> include the recitation of mantras and worship of the demi-gods, who are responsible for helping the individual jiva (person) soul on his/her evolutionary path. These demi-gods are also in charge of the Vedic planets. It may be said that the afflictions here are generalized and do not give an "instant" diagnosis. My response is that, first of all, in allopathic medicine, a diagnosis is given in the terminal stages of the disease, and that labeling is far from "curative." The planetary afflictions, however, can be noted at birth and counseling can be instituted, as well as other Preventative practices of lifestyle modifications, environmental planning and gem therapy. Otherwise, young people frequently develop a casual attitude towards their health, which may result in a "casualty."

Mantra remedies are also extremely valuable, but are not widely practiced in the United States, even though there is widespread knowledge of the efficacy of such practices in the spiritual community. Therefore, gem therapy is widely used in India for relief of planetary afflictions, which lead to spiritual misconceptions, secondly mental aberrations, and thirdly, to physical degenerative states, that are called dis-ease. It is our contention, that if gem therapy is initiated early, and if early spiritual practices are developed (including dietary practices) then dis-ease will not appear, and, if it does appear, it appears in a modified and attenuated form. First, I would like to address the whole topic of color therapy and crystal therapy, about which many books have been written. However, most of these books do not cite any references for their therapeutic effects, a matter that is of great concern to me, since gem therapy is so effective if done properly. For proper guidelines, please check (Planetary Gemnologist Association).

In his book, <u>STELLAR HEALING</u>, N.N. Saha, makes the claim that "gems have wonderful medicinal value in curing dis-eases and they also give protection from dis-eases. They also create immunity in our body against dis-eases. It is also true that gems cannot cure dis-eases like cancer, or cerebral-thrombosis, asthma, etc, but can reduce their effect and give some relief to the victim." In his response to the question "how can gems cure dis-eases?" Saha responds "our body is composed of the seven colors of the rainbow and the Sun has seven colors in its rays. When there is a deficiency of one color, we are attacked with the dis-ease caused by the deficiency of that color. Gems have abundant source of recouping that color into our body and this source is not exhausted even after constant use of several years. Each gem has one color. Suppose when red rays are disturbed or become deficient in our body we suffer from fever, boils, abcesses, carbuncles, etc. and if Red coral is used, on can get relief immediately from such diseases." In his book, ASTROLOGICAL HEALING GEMS, Shivaji Bhattacharjee says "the Science of Astrology involves measuring the subtle forces that pervade the Universe through an understanding of the significance of the various angles adopted by these forces at different times. The claim of astrology is that the subtle cosmic rays, known at the manifest level in terms of seven visible colors and a few invisible rays are the main factors influencing human destiny, effecting our daily and hourly Cycles, and resulting in gradual evolution in the process. If all the phenomenon of the universe are characterized by a wave structure, then there must be a correspondence or resonance between large scale phenomena, such as the cosmic forces, embodied by the planets, and those on a smaller scale, like the human psychological system. "These correspondences have been hinted at in Western occult writings dating back to Ancient times. They occur in Plato, where they appear to have been received from the tradition we call Pythagorean, but which are very likely much older. One basic notion is that there is a Divine Harmony in the Universe which is embodied in the "music of the spheres" and which unites the macrocosm and the microcosm through resonance.

A very important consideration in gem therapy, since it is veritably, a subtle rectification of planetary vibrations, is that the patient's own receptive field be as non-obstructive as possible. Therefore, and in *Ayurveda*, it is a generally accepted practice to follow a strict vegetarian diet. Obviously, such a subtle rectification of cosmic forces via gems requires *" a proper karmic receptive field"* Within the regime of a vegetarian diet, various naturopathic doctors may also prefer subtleties again for rectification of a particular dis-ease (using various spices, etc.) However, this goes beyond my clinical experience and, in that subtle realm, I would simply refer a patient to a naturopath, such as Dr. Arun Sharma, International Institute of Mahayoga and Natural Hygiene.

Dr. Arun Sharma
mahayoga99@gmail.com

REFERENCES:

Dr. Eisenberg's tour of Beijing Medical University with Bill Moyers 1993
http://billmoyers.com/content/the-mystery-of-chi/

Junior Jyotish software http://junior-jyotish.fyxm.net

Planetary Gemonologist Association http://p-g-a.org

***THE SUBJECTIVE EVOLUTION OF CONSCIOUSNESS** by Bhakti Raksak Sridhar dev Goswami, Guardian of Devotion Press, 1989
***HOW TO JUDGE A HOROSCOPE**, B.V. Raman and Gayatri devi Vasudev, IBH Prakashana, 1972
***PRINCIPLES AND PRACTICES OF MEDICAL ASTROLOGY** by Dr. Jagannath Rao, Sagar Publications, New Delhi, 1972
***RAMAN'S 110 YEAR EPHEMERIS OF PLANETARY POSITIONS**, UBSPD Publishers, New Delhi

***ASTRO-LOGOS**, Janes Braha, Hermetician Press, 1989
***THE MERCK MANUAL THIRTEENTH EDITION**, Merck Publishers etal, 1977
***DISPOSITORS IN ASTROLOGY**, J.N. Bhasin, Ranjan Publications, 1982
***MUHURTAS OR ELECTIONAL ASTROLOGY**, B.V. Raman, IBH Prakashana, 1986
***KARMIC ASTROLOGY: THE MOON'S NODES AND REINCARNATION**, Martin Schulman, Publ: Samuel Weiser Inc., York Beach, Maine, 1993
***ALTERNATIVE MEDICINE**, compiled by the Burton Goldberg Group, Future Medicine Publishing, Fife Washington, 1993
***HEALING AND THE MIND**, Bill Moyers in is interview of Dean Ornish, Publ: Doubleday, 1993
***ANATOMY OF THE SPIRIT**, Carolyn Myss, Ph.D, Random House
***BRIHAT PARASARA HORA SHASTRA**, Maharishi Parasara, Ranjan Publications, New Delhi, 1988

*STELLAR HEALING, N.N. Saha, Sagar Publications, New Delhi, 1982cal Healing Gems, Shivaji Battacharajee, Passage Press, Salt Lake City, Utah, 1990

ASTROLOGICAL NATIVES:

You may use the Raman's Ephemeris or a free software called <u>Junior Jyotish</u>
1. Barbara 11/12/1952 @ 10:30 AM
2. Lydia 7/30/1981
3. Machela 8/15/1941
4. Norman 4/21/196@ 12:30 PM, Ill.
5. Ashley 8/30/1986 @ 7:30 AM Fl
6. Margaret 7/13/1971 @ 2:30 PM Ma.
7. Ajah 8/27/1992 NY, NY
8. Cornelia 8/15/1962 Las Vegas, Nev
9. Heidi 11/30/ 1972 @ 5:09 AM, Amherst, Ma.
10. Judy 1/14/1931 @ 3 PM, Pa.
11. Rick W. 9/08/1958, Ashland, Kty
12. Howard A. 12/16/1955, Birmingham, Ala.
13. Gianni Versace 12/02/1946 @ 1:30 PM, Reggio, Di Calabria, italy

14. LYNN 9/02/1956 2 10:57 PM
15. Gato 10/30/1981 @ 0:30 PM, NY, NY
16. Amy 6/24/1979 @ 4:08 AM, Naples, Fl
17. Barbara 6/11/1966, San Francisco, Ca.
18. Lasandra 7/28/1972, Memphis Tn.
19. Allen 9/21/1917, Somerville, Ma.
20. Gudrun C. 2/15/1952 @ 2 AM, Stuttgart, Germany
21. Sue 8/27/1981 2 8:42 am, Cleut, Tx.
22. Naomi 12/19/1951 @ 1:05PM, St. Paul, Mn.
23. Terry B. 12/20/1951 @ 4 AM, NY NY.
24. Denise 1/06/1964@ 12:05 PM
25. Roberta 4/21/1945 @ 8:30 AM, Richmond, Va.
26. Megan 8/11/1977, Va.
27. Melissa 12/19/1978, Wash., D.c.
28. Emma 7/12/1976, Buffalo, NY
29. Jim 6/28/1960, San Francisco, Ca.
30. Joseph T. 11/15/1975
31. Victoria 1/28/1935
32. Herbert M. 6/09/1950, Winterville, N.C.
33. Anna 6/11/1958, Plymouth, Ma.
34. Louise 11/06/1953 @ 6 AM, Hawaii

www.ingramcontent.com/pod-product-compliance
Lightning Source LLC
Chambersburg PA
CBHW031928240526
45464CB00023B/2704